50 Chair Exercises for Seniors;

Relieve Pain, Loss Weight, Improve Balance and Live Longer.

with Pictures and Large Print

Ian Anderson

Copyright © 2020 Ian Anderson

The author of this book does not dispense medical advice or prescribe the use of any technique as a form of treatment for physical, emotional, or medical problems without the advice of a physician, either directly or indirectly. The intent of the author is only to offer information of a general nature to help you in your quest for emotional, physical, and spiritual well-being. In the event you use any of the information in this book for yourself, the author and the publisher assume no responsibility for your actions.

Download Your Free Gift Now

Learn How to

<u>GET Your HEALTH in a Successful Place</u> with Ease!

As a way of saying "thank you" for your purchase, I'm going to share with you a **Free Gift** that is exclusive to readers of "50 Chair Exercises for Seniors; with Pictures and Large Print".

It will help you enjoy your Golden years, improve quality of life, feel more energized!

<u>Click Here to Check it Out</u>

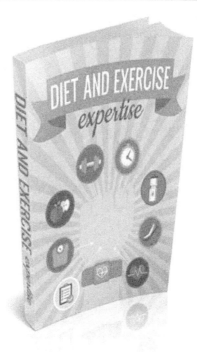

Contents

Introduction

Regular physical activity is key for older adults to experience exercise's physical and mental benefits.

Research evidence supports that engaging in an age-appropriate exercise program can reduce risks of chronic disease, increase life expectancy, maintain functional capacities, and enhance overall physical health.

The American College of Sports Medicine recommends that as long as these fitness programs are tailored to each individual's fitness level the positive benefits of physical activity and exercise can be maximized.

No matter how long it's been since you've kept up with a regular exercise routine, or if you're dealing with the consequences of chronic pain or a disability caused by an accident or health issue, there are still accessible activities that can bolster strength, cardiovascular health, mobility, and balance - all without having to leave your comfortable chair!

Why not give some of these options a try today? With the right plan, you can get back to better fitness in no time.

PART I

Why Chair Exercise?

When you are over the age of 60 you may likely face a unique set of challenges when it comes to finding an effective form of exercise.

Limitations in mobility, balance, and energy can make it difficult to partake in rigorous physical activities; however, chair exercises provide an ideal solution.

Let's take a look at why chair exercises may be the ideal choice for seniors like you.

Low-Impact Workouts

Chair exercises are low-impact workouts that are gentle on joints and muscles.

Low-impact exercises are important when you are older because they reduce the risk of injury and make sure you don't overexert yourself.

With chair exercises, you can still get in a good workout without straining your body or putting unnecessary strain on your joints.

Adaptable to Different Mobility Levels

The beauty of chair exercise is that it can be adapted to different mobility levels. If you have limited mobility due to injury or age-related conditions, you can modify your workout so that it is specifically tailored to meet your needs.

This way, no matter what your physical condition is like, you can find an exercise regimen that works for you!

Variety of Exercises

Finally, there's a wide variety of chair exercises available for seniors over 60. From yoga and strength training to stretching and balance exercises, there's something for everyone!

With so many options available, it's easier than ever to find the perfect routine that works best for your needs and goals.

PART II

What is an Ideal Chair?

Now you know why doing chair exercises is a great way for seniors over 60 to stay in shape and improve their overall health. But what should you look for in an ideal chair for chair exercises?

Let's explore the features of the perfect chair for senior chair exercises so you can make sure you're exercising safely and comfortably.

Safety First

The most important thing to consider when shopping for a chair for your senior chair exercises is safety.

Make sure the legs are securely attached and the arms are sturdy enough to support your weight while exercising.

It's also important to choose a chair with a wide base so that it won't tip over easily.

Lastly, look for a nonslip surface on the seat so you don't slip off while doing your exercises.

Comfort Is Key

Comfort is also very important when doing chair exercises, especially if you plan on using the same chair multiple times each week.

Look for a cushioned seat that won't put too much pressure on your lower back while sitting or exercising, as well as armrests that provide adequate support without digging into your skin.

If possible, try out different chairs before purchasing to make sure it's comfortable enough for regular use.

Size Matters

When choosing an ideal chair, size matters! If you plan on using the same chair multiple times each week, make sure it's not too big or too small for your body type or height.

You want to be able to sit in the seat comfortably with both feet flat on the floor and still have room to move around during your exercises without feeling cramped or restricted in any way.

PART III

When should seniors consider chair exercise?

The American Heart Association recommends that seniors engage in at least 150 minutes of moderate-intensity aerobic activity per week. For those who are unable to stand or walk for long periods, chair exercise can provide an effective alternative way to reach this goal.

Seniors should consider chair exercise if they have any of the following conditions: balance issues, limited mobility due to injury or illness, or restricted range of motion due to age.

Let's take a closer look at some other factors to consider before adopting chair exercises.

Medical Conditions

If you suffer from a medical condition that affects your mobility, such as arthritis, then chair exercise may be the best option for you.

Even if you don't have any medical issues, it's easy for seniors to overdo it with regular exercise and end up with an injury or other issue that could hinder their overall health.

Chair exercises are designed with safety in mind, so they provide low-impact activities that reduce the risk of injury while still providing benefits like improved balance and flexibility.

Joint Pain

Joint pain is another reason why seniors might prefer chair exercises over other forms of physical activity.

Low-impact exercises like these are gentle on the joints and don't require any straining or stretching movements that could cause further discomfort or pain. Chair exercises also help improve joint flexibility, which can help alleviate pain in the long run.

Energy Level

Energy levels can vary day by day as we age; some days you may feel energized enough to go out running while other days may leave you feeling more sluggish than usual.

On those days when energy levels are low, chair exercises can be incredibly beneficial because they require minimal effort but still provide all the benefits of regular physical activity without having to put too much strain on your body.

PART IV
Benefits of Chair Exercise

Improved Flexibility

Performing exercises in a seated position allows seniors to safely stretch their arms and legs without putting too much strain on their joints, muscles, or ligaments.

Through stretching and active movement, seniors can improve their range of motion while also increasing their flexibility. This is especially important as we age since our bodies naturally become less flexible over time.

Increased Strength and Endurance

Chair exercises aren't just about stretching—they can also help you increase the strength in your arms and legs.

Certain exercises like alternating leg lift help strengthen leg muscles while arm curls with resistance bands help tone upper body muscles.

By engaging in these activities regularly, you can also build more muscle mass which will lead to increased energy levels throughout the day.

Improves Balance

Balance issues are common among older adults which increases their risk of falls and other accidents.

Fortunately, chair exercises such as side-stepping movements or heel raises can be used to improve balance over time.

Exercises that involve shifting weight from one side of the body to the other will help improve coordination and stability so seniors feel safer when they're on their feet.

Mental Stimulation

Chair exercise isn't just good for physical health; it offers mental benefits as well! Exercise helps stimulate blood flow to the brain which improves cognitive function and memory recall.

Plus, chair exercises provide a sense of routine and accomplishment which helps fight boredom or feelings of loneliness that may otherwise arise during retirement years.

Promote Overall Health and well-being

Physical activity does more than just keep your body fit—it keeps your mind healthy too! Regular exercise has been shown to reduce stress levels while boosting moods due to endorphin production in the brain when we move our bodies around.

Chair exercise is a safe way for seniors to get moving without risking injury while still reaping all the rewards of regular physical activity like improved sleep quality, better immunity against illness, and stronger bones & joints overall!

PART V
Importance of Stretching

Stretching is one of the most important activities we can do to maintain our physical health. Not only does stretching help reduce the risk of injury, but it can also help improve circulation and flexibility, relieve tension, and even enhance athletic performance.

Regular stretching helps lengthen muscles, allowing them to contract more powerfully following a workout or activity. Additionally, stretching helps to elongate joints and decrease stiffness in the body.

In other words, regular stretching provides a foundation for long-term body function and movement. Stretching should be an integral part of any exercise routine as it helps prevent physical problems stemming from too little movement over time.

Let's look at the different types of stretching.

Static Stretching

Static stretching is the most common type of stretching. This involves slowly extending a muscle to its maximum point and holding it for 30 seconds or more to increase flexibility and reduce tension.

Static stretching is best done after warming up with light activity such as walking or jogging to raise your body temperature and make the muscles more pliable.

It's important to take your time when performing static stretching exercises — never force yourself into positions that cause pain or discomfort.

Dynamic Stretching

Dynamic stretching is an active form of stretching that uses movement to increase flexibility. This type of stretching requires you to move through ranges of motion while simultaneously working on balance and coordination.

Dynamic stretches are great for seniors because they help improve mobility while engaging multiple muscle groups at once. Examples include leg swings, arm circles, hip circles, high kicks, and lunge walks.

Proprioceptive Neuromuscular Facilitation (PNF) Stretching

PNF stretching is a type of dynamic stretching that combines passive and active movements with muscular contractions to improve range-of-motion (ROM).

This type of stretch engages both the agonist muscles (the prime movers) and antagonist muscles (the antagonists) to create a stronger ROM than other forms of dynamic stretches alone could provide.

PNF stretches should be performed with care as they can put a strain on joints if not done properly.

How Often Should You Stretch?

As a senior, it's recommended that you stretch your muscles several times a week to prevent stiffness and promote improved comfort and well-being. With each session, make sure to gently move your joints through their full range of motion and hold stretches for around 15 seconds.

Try to focus on areas like the neck, shoulders, back, hips, knees, and ankles; these areas need extra attention in older adults since stiffness and aches seem to accumulate there over time.

Timing Your Stretches

As far as timing goes, you should aim for 10 minutes of stretching per day to reap the full benefits.

This can be done all at once or split up into two 5-minute sessions throughout the day - whichever works best with your schedule! However, if you're feeling any excess pain or discomfort while stretching then take a break and consult your doctor before continuing any routine.

Now that you know the basics and benefits of chair exercises, let's explore how you should warm up.

PART VI

Warm-Up

Neck Stretch

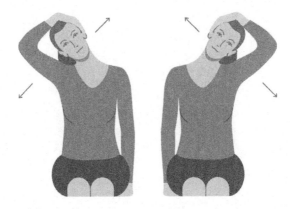

A seated neck stretch is an ideal way to keep your upper body mobile and supple as you gradually stretch and release the tension in your neck muscles.

Firstly, sit in a chair with good posture ensuring your back is supported at all times.

Next, tilt your head towards the right shoulder before holding the pose for 15 - 30 seconds and then slowly coming back to the center.

Do the same thing on the left shoulder side and repeat on each side three times. Remember - keep breathing during the process and don't rush any steps!

Seated Shoulder Circles

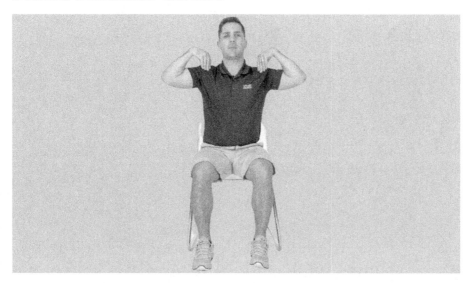

Start by sitting up comfortably in a sturdy chair with both feet firmly on the ground. Make sure that your back is straight and lifted chest high.

Then, place your fingertips gently on either side of the tops of your shoulders.

Finally, start moving your arms in small circles outwards and upwards for about 10 reps before reversing the motion for another 10 reps.

Seated Back Bend

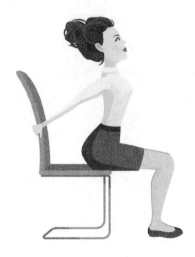

Start by sitting on the edge of your seat with feet hip distance apart, legs slightly turned out with soles flat on the ground.

Keep your spine in its natural C shape while your hands hold on to the back of the chair and keep your head in line with your spine.

Your weight should be evenly distributed right through your arms, shoulders, back, and chest as you slowly begin to lean backward.

The aim is to extend the spine carefully yet confidently feeling a gentle stretch along your upper body.

As far back as feels comfortable, hold the posture whilst breathing normally and relaxing tension away from any tight spots before slowly returning to an upright position.

Neck Rolls

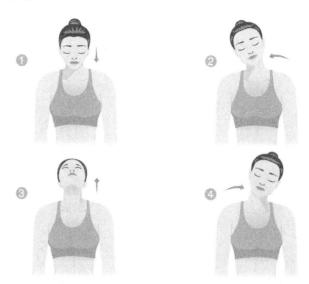

Begin by sitting tall with your chin level with the ground, then slowly tilt your head to one side so that it is resting on your shoulder while keeping both shoulders relaxed on the ground (do not lift them).

Hold this position for 5 seconds before returning to center and repeating on the other side of your neck; complete 3 sets of 10 reps on each side of the neck (20 total reps).

This helps increase flexibility in both sides of the neck as well as helps to reduce tension headaches due to poor posture or stress throughout the day.

Seated Overhead Stretch

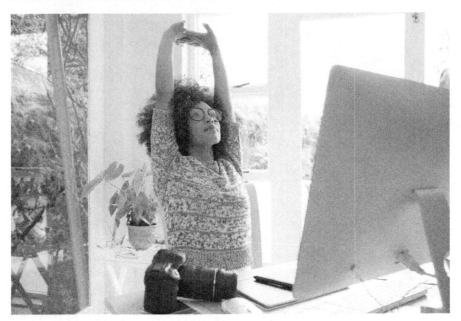

To begin, sit upright with your feet together and arms by your side.

Gently reach up with your interlocked fingers towards the ceiling and hold for 10 to 20 seconds.

You should feel a stretch in your abdominal muscles.

Hip Flexor Stretch

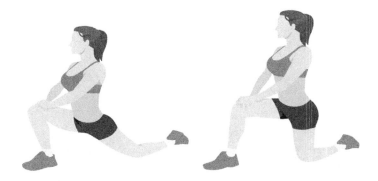

Assume a kneeling position on your yoga mat or exercise mat, with your bottom positioned on the heels of your feet and the balls of your feet, pressed firmly against the mat.

Gradually lean forward, and move your palms to rest on the ground - hands should be kept shoulder width apart, and elbows bent to prevent them from locking.

To stretch out further, move your left knee forward into the gap between your arms, ensuring that the left foot is firmly planted flat onto the floor in front of you to create a 90-degree angle.

Place both hands on top of your left knee for balance and support before extending the right leg behind you; make sure that both knee and foot are pressed firmly onto the mat.

Slightly lean forward to feel a deeper stretch throughout, hold it for 20-30 seconds then release.

Seated Chest Exercises

Seated Chest Flys

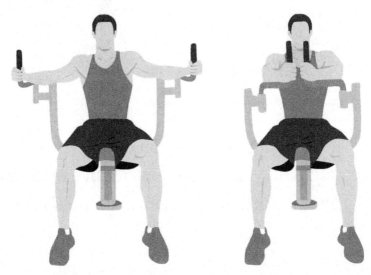

To begin, sit upright in a chair with both feet flat on the ground and hold a light weight in each hand with palms facing forward away from your body.

Inhale deeply while extending both arms out wide at shoulder level before slowly bringing them together again directly over your chest while exhaling fully.

Pause here for 2-3 seconds before returning to the starting position with arms out wide again at shoulder level while inhaling fully once more—repeat this 8-12 times for 2 -3 sets.

Seated Push-Ups

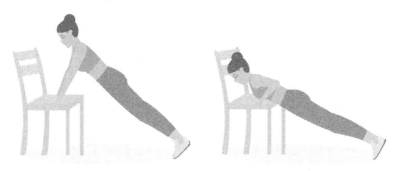

Place both hands firmly against the seat of the chair at shoulder level before taking your feet backward until you feel the weight on your upper body.

Once ready, inhale deeply then slowly bend elbows outward until they form 90-degree angles before pushing yourself back up into starting position while exhaling fully—repeat this 10 - 15 times for 2 - sets.

Seated Chest Press

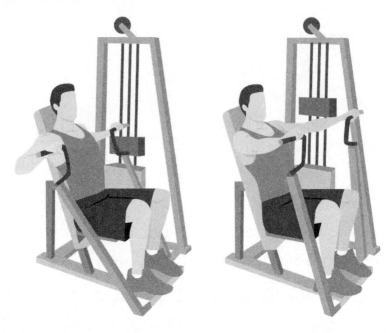

Start by sitting in an armless chair with back support, and hold a weight in each hand with palms facing forward.

Your arms should be slightly bent at the elbows, and keep them level with your shoulders as you simultaneously press the weights away from your chest.

Breathe out as you push away from your chest and keep your elbows close to your body for maximum effect.

As you bring them back in, breathe in through your nose, and repeat for the desired number of repetitions.

Chair Exercises For Shoulders

Shoulder Rotations

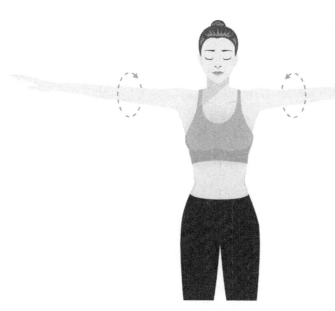

Begin by sitting or standing upright with feet flat on the ground and holding onto weights or just use your hands if not available.

Start by raising both arms outwards at chest level then rotate them left to right 10 times before switching directions (right-left) for another 10 times on each side (for a total of 20 rotations).

Lateral Raise

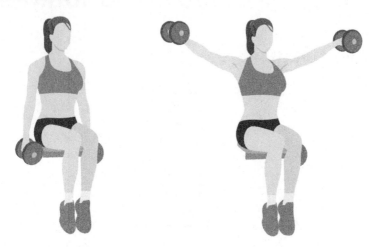

Begin by sitting down in a chair with your back straight and feet firmly on the floor. With a light weight in each hand and palms facing forward, slowly lift both arms out to the side until they are parallel with the floor.

Hold this position for two or three seconds before slowly lowering your arms back down to the starting position.

It's important to keep your elbows slightly bent throughout the exercise, as fully extended arms can put a strain on the shoulder joint.

Aim for 2 - 3 sets of 8-12 repetitions, per session, increasing the weight over time as you gain strength and become more comfortable with the movement pattern.

Seated Shoulder Press

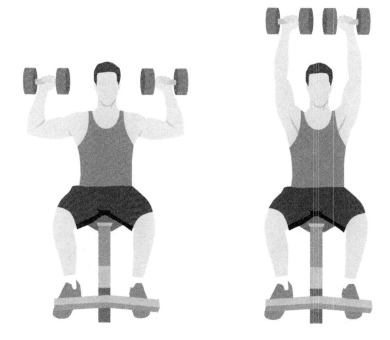

Put your feet flat on the floor and sit with your back straight. Start with your arms relaxed at shoulder level and hold one of the weights in each hand.

Slowly exhale as you push the weight upwards until your arms become straight but not locked out.

Then slowly return the weights to shoulder level while inhaling.

Be mindful of maintaining a controlled motion throughout the exercise so that tension stays steady and even on both sides of your body. Perform 2 - 3 sets of 10 - 12 repetitions.

Seated Front Raises

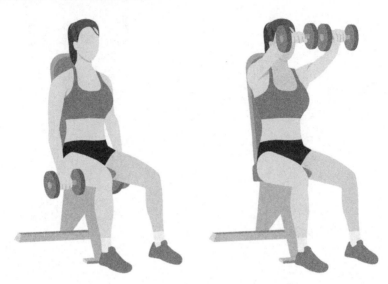

To properly perform the move, begin by sitting on a sturdy bench or chair with no arms. Keep your chest up tall, shoulders down, and back and abs engaged.

Start with light dumbbells in each hand with your palms facing away from you and elbows relaxed so they're equal with your shoulder.

As you exhale, press the dumbbells up until they reach just above your shoulders, and then inhale as you bring them back to the starting position.

Make sure that during this exercise you are keeping your core tight, making no jerky movements with the arms, and focusing on proper form over speed.

Seated Upright Row

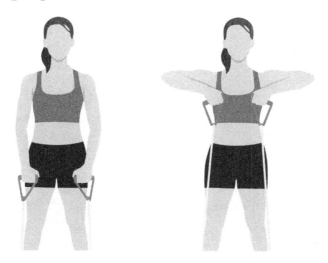

Begin by sitting or standing upright with a weight or resistance band in hand placed just below waistline level.

Start pulling both hands up towards the armpit area while keeping elbows up high together throughout the entire motion level before slowly lowering them back down again towards starting position.

Repeat this motion for 10-15 reps for 2 - 3 sets.

Chair Exercises for Arms

Bicep Curls

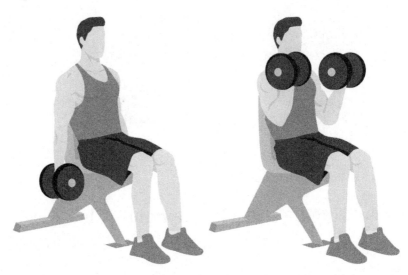

To begin, sit with your back firmly against a backrest so that your head and shoulders make complete contact with the surface. Make sure your feet are solidly on the ground.

Once you are comfortable, grasp your dumbbell or resistance bands with your palms facing forward and wrap your thumbs around the handles.

Hold them close to your body. Simultaneously depress and retract your shoulder blades for support.

When performing the upward phase of this exercise, it is important to exhale slowly and bend both elbows at the same time, bringing the dumbbells close to your chest without arching your back or excessively extending your elbows.

Keep a neutral wrist position throughout the lift and keep contact with your head and shoulders against the bench while pressing your butt firmly against it.

Your feet should remain planted firmly in place on the floor, avoiding any shoulder shrugs while retracting and depressing your scapulae (shoulders).

During the downward phase of this exercise, remember to take an inhale as you gently lower the dumbbells back to starting position. Performing 2-3 sets of 10 - 12 repetitions is appropriate.

Seated Triceps Extension

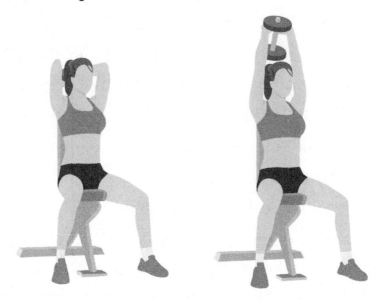

This exercise works your triceps, deltoids, and upper back muscles.

To get started, find a lightweight dumbbell and sit in an upright position. Hold the weight above your head with arms extended and elbows close together.

Now, lower the weight behind you until your elbows come just above shoulder height. Hold this position for 1 -2 seconds before returning to starting position.

Repeat 10 times for 3 sets with 30 - 90 seconds rest between sets.

Tricep Chair Dips

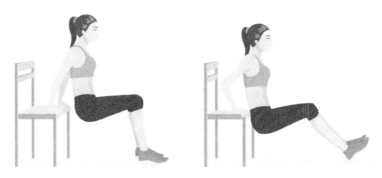

Begin by sitting on the edge of a stable chair, weight bench, or step and firmly gripping the sides adjacent to your hips.

Allow your legs to extend outwards, hip-width apart with your heels resting securely on the ground. Keeping your chin lifted, gaze forward.

Using pressure from your palms as leverage, lift yourself so that your backside is hovering above the chair's edge before slowly lowering until you feel a comfortable bend in your elbows at an angle of 90 degrees.

Throughout this full range of motion strive to move in a controlled manner before pushing yourself back up to almost straight arms and repeating 2 - 3 sets of 10 - 15 repetitions.

Chair Exercises for Back

Shoulder Blade Squeezes

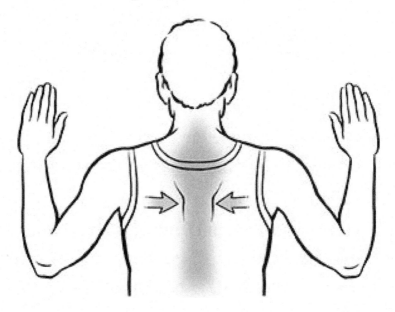

Sit up straight in a chair with your feet flat on the ground. Lift both hands in the air next to your shoulders.

Push your hands behind to feel the tension in both shoulders and upper back muscles, then slowly release them to return to starting position.

Do this exercise 10 times for two sets.

Lat Pulldowns

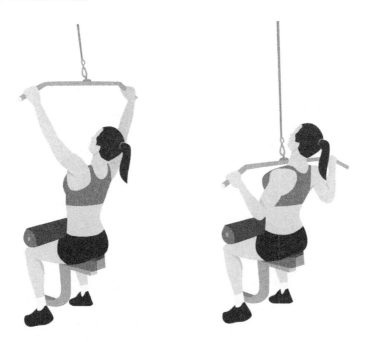

Sit up straight reach above with both hands and grasp onto a resistance band or towel that's attached above head level (like an overhead bar).

Keeping arms extended above head level, pull band/towel down towards chest level until it touches the top of chest; pause for one second before slowly releasing it back up until arms are fully extended again (this is one rep). Do this exercise 10 - 12 times for two sets.

Reverse Flys

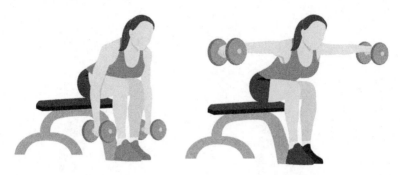

Bring your body forward until you form a bent angle. Hold a pair of light dumbbells (2-5 lbs) in each hand at arm's length next to you, palms facing each other and elbows slightly bent.

Keeping arms straight, lift both arms out to either side until they're parallel with the ground, feeling a pull across upper back muscles as you do so; pause for one second before slowly returning them to starting position. Do this exercise 10 times for two sets.

Seated Row

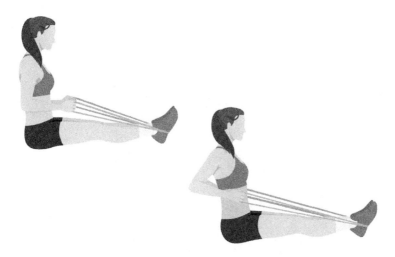

To do the exercise, begin by sitting at the edge of a chair or bench comfortably while fully extending your knee forward.

Grab your resistance band and wrap it around your feet. Keep your core engaged throughout the exercise while pivoting from the hips.

Next, drive your elbows back towards your sides while squeezing your shoulder blades together until the arms are bent.

Return to the starting point with a slow and controlled motion, keeping tension in the muscles throughout each repetition.

 Repeat for 8 to 12 reps for 3 sets as needed. Always remember to use proper technique when performing any exercise for optimal safety and results!

Bent Over Row

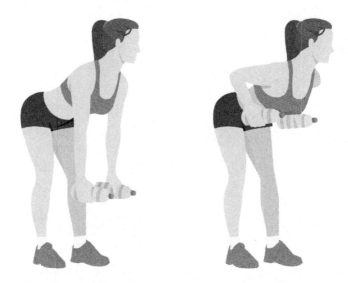

This exercise works the arms, upper back, and shoulder muscles all at once by focusing on pulling movements instead of pushing ones like arm circles or shoulder presses to do.

To begin, sit or stand with good posture while holding two dumbbells or two household objects close together near your chest with palms facing inward toward each other.

Slowly lean forward from the waist until you feel resistance in your core then pull up using only your arms until elbows reach shoulder level again before lowering them back down slowly for 10 repetitions for two sets.

Chair Exercises for Legs

Single Leg knee Extension

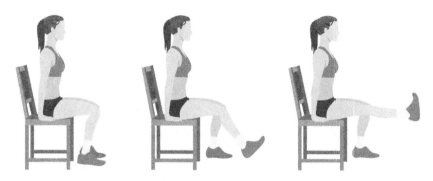

Sit on a chair with your back straight and your chin slightly tucked in. Make sure both feet are flat on the floor.

Place your hands lightly by your sides to provide stability if needed or keep them on your lap if that is more comfortable.

Lift one leg slowly, bringing it out straight while keeping the other foot firmly planted on the ground.

Hold this position for 5 seconds and then slowly lower it back down to its starting position.

Repeat up to 10 times per leg before switching sides and completing any additional repetitions with your other leg as desired.

Calf Raises

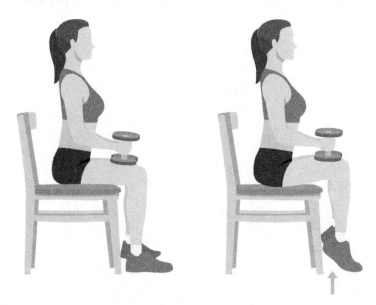

To get maximum benefit, be sure to sit up tall in a chair with your feet firmly planted on the floor and apart at a hip distance.

With your core engaged and eyes facing forward, lift one foot as high as you can onto your toes while engaging your calf muscles.

Lower the heel back to the ground in a controlled manner and repeat 10 times before switching to the other leg.

Three sets of 10 reps per leg should suffice; however, you can try one additional set with both feet lifting together at the same time, ending with holding both heels up for 10 seconds each.

Sit-and-stands

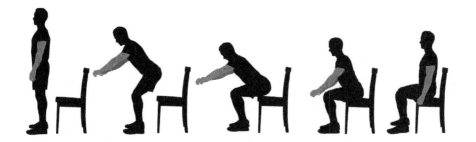

To start, it's important to find a sturdy chair and plant the feet on the floor, about hip distance apart.

You must use as little assistance from their hands or arms as possible when completing this exercise.

Engaging the core, tip forward from the hips before pressing your weight through all four corners of your feet and standing up, extending both the knees and hips fully.

Then repeat the movement by pressing your hips back and carefully bending the knees to return to a seated position.

If you're having difficulty rising to a standing position, start by shifting your weight forward and lifting your glutes just a couple of inches off the chair seat.

Once you reach that height, hold it for one second before slowly lowering back down.

Modified Squats

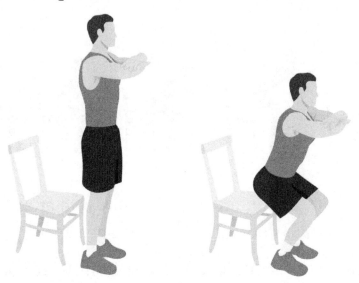

This relatively low-impact exercise helps build muscle while reducing strain on the joints.

To begin, find a chair with a backrest and seat that are both padded.

Stand in front of the chair with feet hip-width apart. Ensure that your toes point away from your body.

You can grip the armrest or fold your hand at your chest level.

Slowly bend your knees while lowering yourself into a seated position stopping only when your thighs are parallel to the floor.

Then, press firmly down through your feet as you lift yourself back up to standing, straightening your legs fully before releasing your grip from the armrests.

Aim for 3 sets of 8 - 12 repetitions for best results, with short, rests in between each set as needed.

Seated Abductions

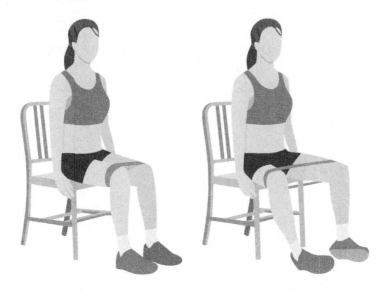

Sit down in the chair, with feet hip-distance apart on the floor. Place the middle of the band around your legs, just under your knees.

Holding onto both ends of the band, slowly open and close your legs, keeping tension on the band at all times.

Make sure to keep your back upright and shoulders relaxed while you do this move. Repeat 10-15 times for 2 sets.

Modified Leg Lifts

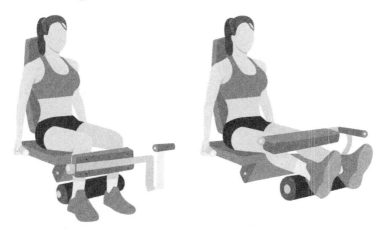

Get into a seated position by making sure your hips, shoulders, and neck are aligned with perfect posture.

Secure your place in the chair by holding onto the armrests or gripping the seat.

Take a deep breath in, then lift both legs as you exhale (with bent knees) until they reach as high as possible.

Hold this position for 5 seconds before releasing it back down to the ground. Do 10-12 repetitions while slowly increasing the number of sets to 3-5.

Tip Toeing

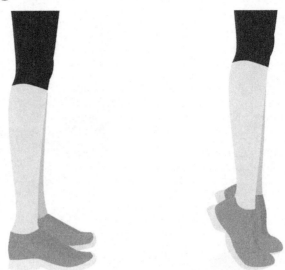

Sit on a chair with knees bent and feet flat on the floor. Make sure your back is straight and your chin is tucked in slightly.

Place your index fingers lightly against the wall in front of you at shoulder height, with your arms slightly bent at the elbows.

Slowly raise your heels onto your tiptoes, using your fingertips to provide support if needed. Hold this position for 10 seconds while drawing your abdominal muscles inward toward your spine without arching or curving the lower back.

Release back down to starting position slowly and repeat 8-10 times or until fatigued.

Seated Heel Slides

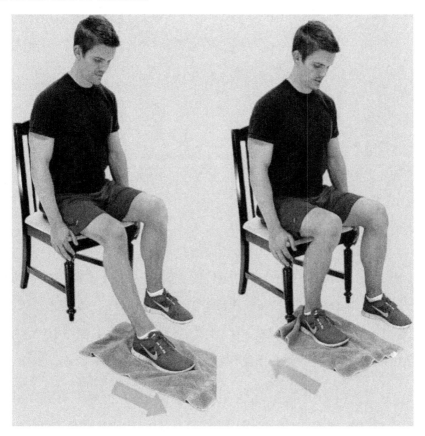

Your foot should be placed on a towel that is on the floor. Move your leg forward slowly before sliding it back to the starting position.

Keep your upper body still and gently engage core muscles; this will help keep you from overextending yourself.

You can do this for 10 reps of 2 sets. Once you become comfortable with this move, you can increase repetitions for a more vigorous exercise routine.

Standing leg curls

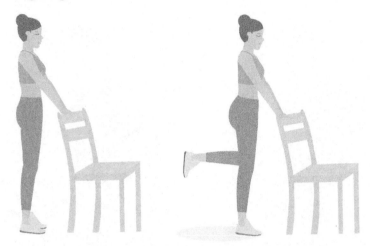

Begin by standing behind a chair and grasping the back for support. Facilitate stability by shifting your weight onto your left leg and gently bending the right knee, bringing your heel towards the buttocks.

Ensure that both legs maintain a slight bend during the curl before slowly returning to the starting position. Alternate legs for 12 to 15 repetitions for 2 - 3 sets.

Chair Exercises for Core

Seated Torso Twists

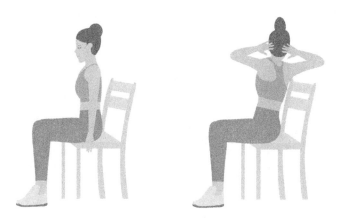

To complete this exercise, begin by sitting with a straight back on the edge of a chair.

Place your feet firmly on the ground and make sure your spine is aligned with the top of your head reaching towards the ceiling.

Next, slowly rotate your upper body to the right side while keeping your lower body in place.

Hold this position for 10 seconds and take several deep breaths.

Afterward, repeat on the left side and hold it for another 10 seconds before returning to a neutral position.

As you do this exercise be mindful not to arch or sway too far in either direction as these movements can cause strain on muscles near your spine if done incorrectly. Ideally, you should do 2-3 sets of this exercise.

Modified Planks

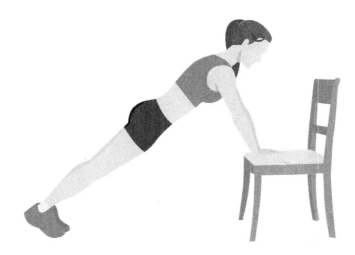

To utilize the chair modification of the plank, use the seat of the chair

Start by placing your hands firmly on the seat of your chair, keeping them shoulder-distance apart.

Step back until your body forms a slanted line from head to heel. Keep your arms straight, and hips aligned between your knees and shoulders, and focus on working your abs to stay steady.

Hold for 10 to 60 seconds before returning to an upright position.

Do three sets, and increase time with each set as you become more comfortable holding the plank without any drop in form.

Knee Lifts

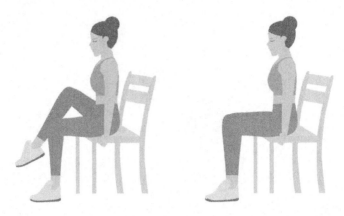

Start by sitting up tall in a chair with feet flat on the floor about shoulder-width apart, and hands placed lightly on kneecaps (optional).

Keeping both feet planted firmly on the ground, lift one knee towards the chest while keeping the upper body stable throughout the movement (avoid leaning too far forward).

Hold knee against chest before slowly lowering back down into starting position then repeat the process with another knee.

Perform 10-15 reps per leg before returning to the starting position. You can do 2-3 sets of this.

Seated Half Roll-Backs

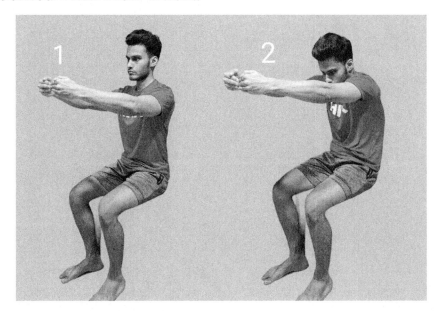

Sit in a comfortable position with your feet on the ground and your knees bent.

Create a circle with your arms in front of your chest. As you do this, be sure to maintain an upright posture.

Now, concentrate on gently curving your spine backward - imagine scooping in the abdominals as you go.

Once you can't move any further, take a slow and steady breath while engaging your core to return the body to its starting position.

Slow and controlled movements are key when performing this exercise to properly tone and shape the body. 2 sets of 10 -12 reps are recommended.

Seated Side Bends

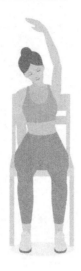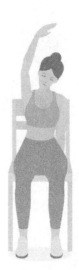

The perfect way to stretch your side is to start by sitting with your knees bent and your feet firmly planted.

Bend your right arm at the elbow and bring it up toward the right side of your head.

With your left arm hanging at your side and maintaining an upright posture free of slouching or leaning back, it's time to get started.

Take a deep breath in, then slowly exhale while gently bending forward from the waist and lowering your left arm towards the floor.

Your chest should be kept open as you carefully pull back on your right elbow for that right-side stretch.

Slowly inhale once more as you rise back into starting position and repeat to complete one cycle. You can do this for two sets of 10 reps.

Chair Aerobics for Cardio

Seated Jumping Jacks

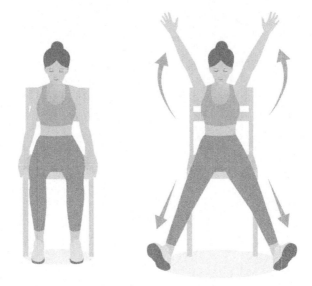

Start by sitting up straight in a chair, with your feet on the floor and knees together.

Point your toes outwards and make sure your arms are bent at the elbows and open to the sides, palms facing forwards.

Lift both legs to the side and flex your feet as you move them outwards, landing on your heels.

Bring your arms together above your head like a regular jumping jack before returning to your starting position.

Repeat 25-30 times in succession.

Seated Skater Switch

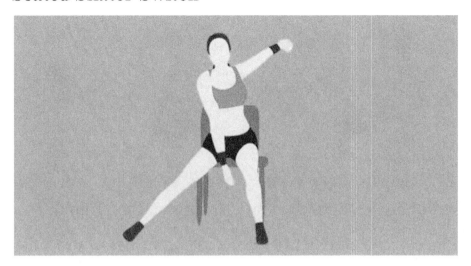

Start by sitting down and extending your legs out in front of you. Make sure to keep your back straight and raise your arms above your head.

Then, have one leg slightly bent at the knee and the other extending away from the body.

Now, take those raised arms and alternately switch sides by moving each arm across to opposite sides of the body as if you are skating.

With each side switch make sure to move slowly and gently; that way you won't strain any muscles or ligaments.

Seated Knee Tucks

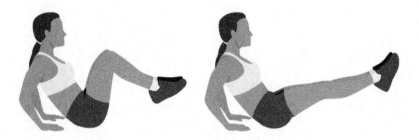

To perform this exercise, begin by sitting in a chair with your feet comfortably resting on the ground.

Place your hands either behind you or off to the sides for support. Tighten your abdominal muscles and hinge at the hips as you draw both knees toward your chest while keeping them bent.

Hold this position for a few seconds then return your feet to the starting point. Repeat 10-20 times or as many repetitions as you feel comfortable with before taking a break.

Leg Lift and Twist

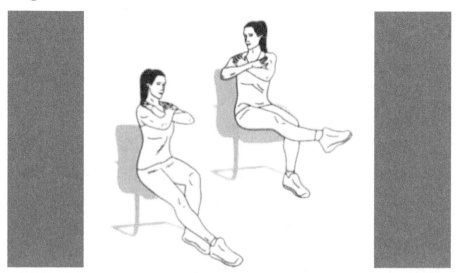

Start by sitting on the edge of a chair and extending your right leg out straight in front while keeping your foot firmly grounded. Then, move to cross arms over the chest area with abs engaged tight.

Now it's time to rotate your torso towards the right as you lift the extended right leg to meet the opposing left knee.

Make sure to press your knees together during this step before returning to the original starting position.

Finally, switch sides and repeat! Aim for 15- 25 of these reps for maximum effect.

Hinge And Cross

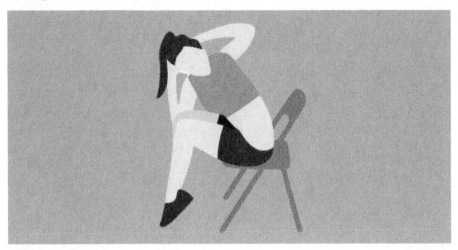

Start by sitting up straight in a chair with your knees together and toes pointed.

Then lift your hands behind your head and focus on bracing your abdominal muscles. Hinge back slightly so that your shoulder blades are just grazing the back of the chair.

Now, cross your right elbow over to touch the left knee, then return to the starting position before switching sides and repeating this motion 20 times.

Flexibility Exercises in a Sitting Position

Back Extension

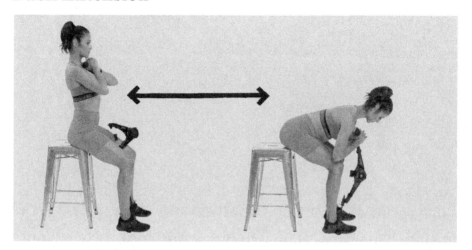

Start by sitting back in your chair with your back positioned securely against the backrest. Rest the palms of your hands on your chest, then lean gently back over the chair back.

You'll feel a soothing stretch across your upper body as you gradually relax this way for 10-15 seconds.

Hamstring Stretch

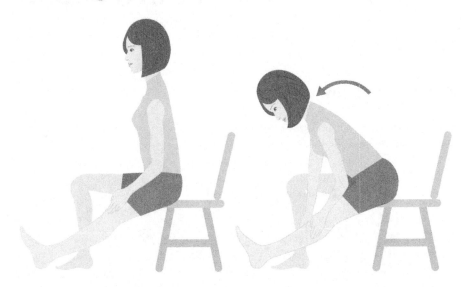

Place your feet flat on the floor and engage your core to stabilize yourself as you bring one foot forward until it's fully stretched.

Have both hands on the knee of this leg; keep your back straight and maintain an upright posture as you gently press down into that top leg for 15 seconds then switch leg positions and repeat.

As you feel comfortable, you can also deepen the stretch by leaning forward and reaching toward your toes.

Hip Stretch

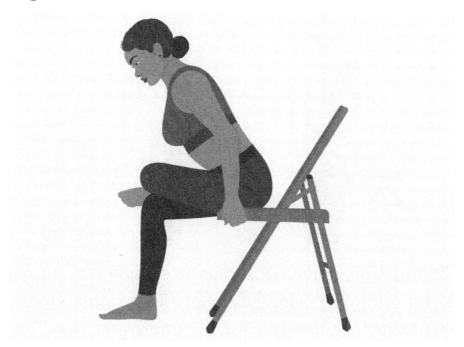

When seated, cross your left ankle over the right knee while maintaining a tall posture.

After than slowly bring your upper body forward to get a stretch through the right glute.

To help intensify the impact, lean forward until you can touch your ankles and hold this position for 15 seconds before moving onto the other side.

Wrist Stretch

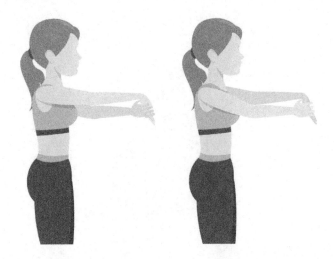

Start by extending your right arm straight out in front of you with your palm facing up. Flexing your wrist so that your fingertips are pointed towards the floor, use your left hand to carefully pull back on your fingers until you feel a stretch along your arm.

Make sure to hold this stretch for 15 seconds before switching sides and repeating the process, then complete the exercise with both arms by repeating the same movements with your palm facing down and fingers flexing upwards.

Seated Shoulder Openers

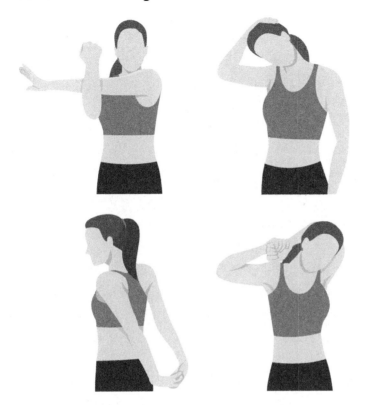

To perform shoulder openers while sitting, sit up straight with both feet flat on the ground and clasp both hands together behind your head, elbows pointing outward.

From here, gently push your elbows backward until you feel a gentle stretch across your chest and shoulders. Hold this position for 10-20 seconds before releasing.

Chest stretch

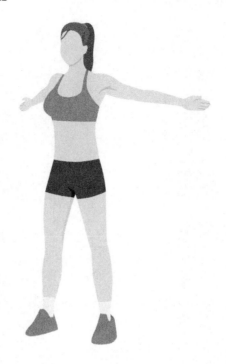

To get started, stand or sit up straight with your feet flat on the floor and shoulder-width apart.

Then, reach both arms out to your sides so your palms are facing forward. Exhale as you slowly draw your arms back together, squeezing your shoulder blades together for 10-30 seconds of a hold.

Afterward, relax and return to the starting position. Repeat this 3-5 times for best results.

Seated Forward Bend

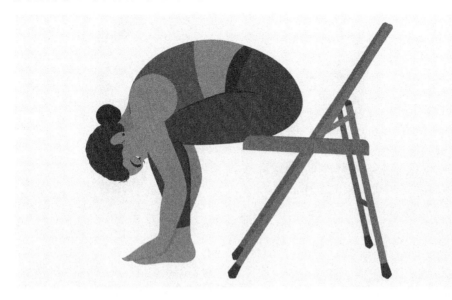

Begin by sitting on a chair with your feet flat on the floor, hip-distance apart. Make sure you have plenty of space around you to stretch out. Take a deep breath, and then slowly exhale as you lean forward from the hips.

As you lean forward focus on reaching toward your toes or the floor. When stretching make sure to never force your body beyond its limit, but rather hold the stretch at a comfortable tension that is still challenging both physically and mentally.

You can hold this pose for up to 15 - 30 seconds before experimenting with other variations of seated forward bends such as grabbing onto your feet.

Cat/Cow Stretch

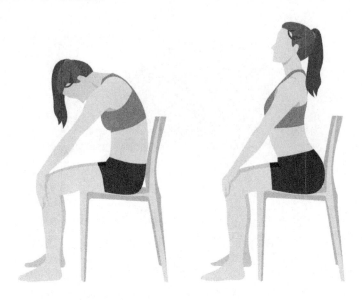

To perform this stretch while sitting, start by sitting up tall with feet planted firmly on the ground about hip-width apart (feet should be parallel).

From here, arch your back slightly (like a cat) then round it forward (like a cow) continuing between these two poses 8-10 times before releasing from the pose completely.

Spinal Twist

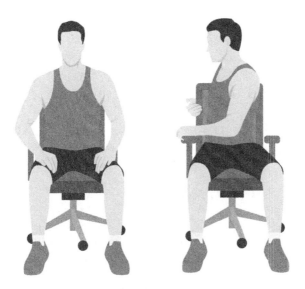

Sit with your feet placed flat on the floor and engage your abdominal muscles.

Gently start to rotate your torso to the right - you can use your left hand to hold the outside of your right knee, for greater stability, while placing the other hand on either the armrest or seat back for further support.

Remember to relax and go only as far as you are comfortable - small rotations can make a big difference. Sustain this stretch for 15-30 seconds and then switch sides.

Congrats! Note from the Author / Publisher:

You've reached the end of the book!

Thank you for finishing 50 Chair Exercises for Seniors; with Pictures and Large Print!

Looks like you enjoyed it!

If so, would you mind taking 30 seconds to leave a quick review on Amazon?

We worked hard to bring you books that you enjoy!

Plus, it helps authors like us produce more books like this in the future!

Here's where to go to leave a review now:

{YOUR BOOK PAGE DIRECT LINK}

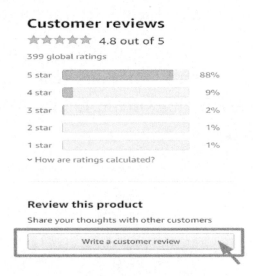

Printed in Great Britain
by Amazon

44667730R00046